“If it doesn’t challenge you, it won’t change you.”

-Unknown

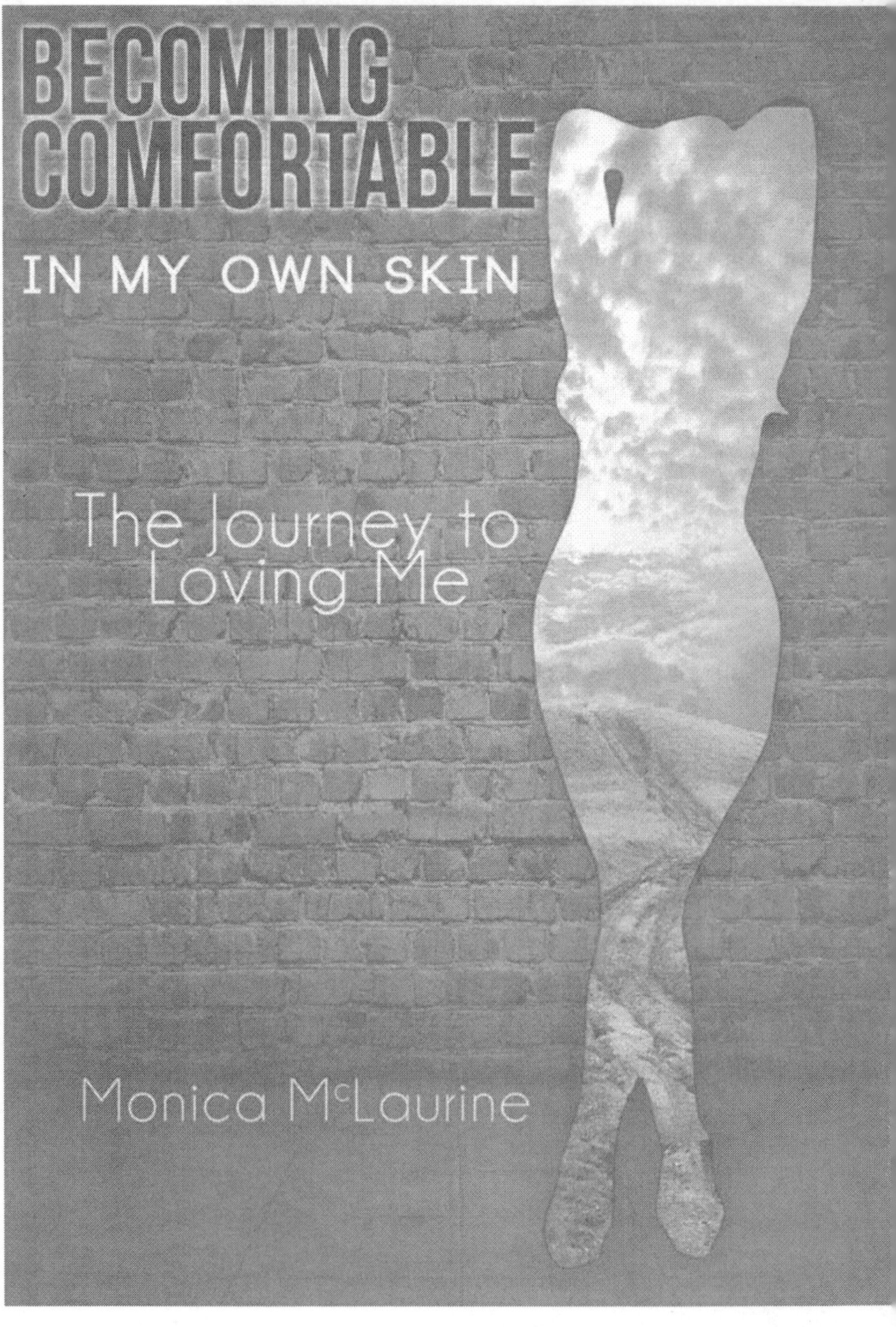
BECOMING
COMFORTABLE
IN MY OWN SKIN
The Journey to
Loving Me
Monica McLaurine

For information contact: MRenee Enterprise Inc.
P.O. Box 694
LaVergne, TN 37086
Website : mmclaurine.com
Email : monica@mmclaurine.com

Book and Cover design by Tonya Osborne of Osborne Photo and Design

Printed in the United States of America

ISBN: 978-0-692-43580-9

LCCN: 2015907167

*This Book is Dedicated to three special women…….*

# *My Guardian Angels*

*My Beloved Grandmother*

## Catherine "Cat" Lytle

*My Sweet Granny*

## Joann Robertson

*My Anointed Cousin*

## La'Kisha Mitchell

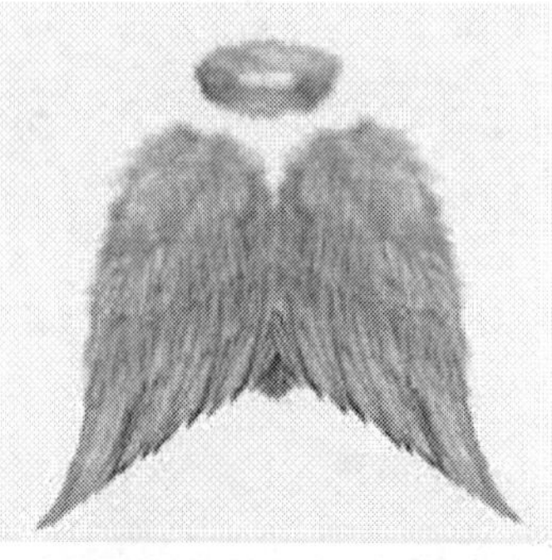

## A Note of Heart-filled Thanks......

First, I must give thanks to my Lord and Savior for entrusting me with this vision to share with the world. I know I was hesitant at first, but thank you for your continued guidance to show me one of my purposes in life. Heart-felt thanks go out to my family for always supporting me, no matter what. Your encouragement and love is priceless to me, and I am forever grateful to you all. Thank you to Pastor John and Lady Alethia Faison, and the Watson Grove Missionary Baptist Church, the best church this side of heaven. Thank you for believing in me, and your willingness to invest in me. I am eternally grateful for your generosity. Last, but certainly not least, to all of my many supporters, thank you for your constant support and encouragement. I don't know what I would do without you all. I love you all to life!

# Table of Contents

# Preface

Through its ups and downs my journey continues to be worth every minute........

## My Journey Starts Here

First, let me say thank you for taking the time out to read my book. You could have done a number of things in your spare time, but you chose to spend it reading my story. For that, I am eternally grateful.

Now, let's get to the reason for this book. There was a time in my life where I always had a smile on my face. I looked like I had it all together and never had a care in the world. I always made sure that I looked well put together, from head to toe. Yeah, I was overweight, but I was tall and shapely, so I could get away with the extra weight sometimes. I presented myself as if nothing was ever wrong, and as if I was on cloud nine all the time. Well, let me let you in on a little secret, I was so unhappy. I had low self-esteem. I would try to dress myself up to mask how I was really feeling. I loved being there for others, but I was so busy being there for them, and helping them with their issues, that it gave me an excuse not to deal with my own.

I struggled with my weight throughout my adult life. If you have ever been overweight then you know how cruel people can be. I never addressed the effects of the hurtful and downright mean things they would say to me. On the outside, I acted as if those statements didn't hurt me, but on the inside, my heart was being ripped out. I just thought if I ignored it, or acted like it didn't bother me, it would stop. I just kept burying it and never dealt with it. Let me share this with you: ignoring your hurt is a very detrimental thing to do. You cannot heal anything that you do not acknowledge. You need to address it. Ignoring my issues earlier in life caused them to come back to haunt me in my adult life.

As I stated earlier, my weight was something I struggled with as I got older. Well, one day, one picture changed the course of my life. I finally decided that enough was enough, and I was going to do something about my weight once and for all. Little did I know that embarking on this journey was going to change my life forever.

Once I started on my journey, I was in the zone. I was so determined that I lost twenty-four pounds in less than two months. I was so excited! I was so proud of myself! I was accomplishing my goal of losing weight. Well, while I was so caught up in the excitement of losing weight, I heard God speak to me, telling me to share my story. I remember thinking, "Lord, I am too embarrassed to tell my story. I just don't want to tell anyone." Well, once I got off of my pity bus I decided to be obedient. On June 3, 2013 I told my abbreviated story on Facebook. I had no idea that sharing my story would have such a significant impact. I had so many likes, response posts, inbox messages, phone calls and text messages. I was very overwhelmed by the support I received from family, friends and strangers alike. They were not only supportive, but were also asking me for help and encouragement. It was at that moment that I understood why God wanted me to share my story. I am just like everyone else. If others could see me losing weight they knew they could do it as well. They were looking at me as an inspiration. What? Are you serious!?! Me? I have always believed that God can use anyone, so why not me? So, in this moment I found my purpose. I couldn't believe that I was inspiring others. Not only that, they were inspiring me as well. They were keeping me accountable. I will talk about the importance of accountability a little later on.

Also, while I was going through my weight loss, I took the opportunity to deal with some old issues that I had buried. It was not easy, but it had to be done. I knew if I was to continue my journey, I had to address all of those hurt feelings and insecurities. It was hard going through the process, but I am so glad I did. I am better for it. So many times when we do not address our past hurts and issues, we hinder our growth. I am determined to continue my mental and spiritual growth and will do what is necessary to make this happen.

As you read this book, you will see my journey and the transparency in which I am sharing my story. I am prayerful that it will help others as they go through their own journeys. Be encouraged and never give up!

# Reflection

1. Have you ever struggled with your weight? If so, explain.

_______________________________________________

_______________________________________________

_______________________________________________

2. Do you have any unresolved issues that you need to deal with? If so, what are they?

_______________________________________________

_______________________________________________

_______________________________________________

Notes:

_______________________________________________

_______________________________________________

_______________________________________________

_______________________________________________

# Chapter 1

~Self~awareness is priceless...

Recognize when it is time for a change. ~

Monica McLaurine

## The Day My Life Changed

March 19, 2013 is the day that changed my life. I was attending a baby shower/birthday party to celebrate with some friends of mine. I can remember it as if it were yesterday. I had on a new outfit, and I thought I was so cute (I was, but stay with me). I had gotten the shirt from a local boutique, and I bought some leggings to go with it. I looked in the mirror and I was pleased. I was dressed to kill and ready to have some fun. A really good friend came to town for this event and we all wanted to get as many pictures of each other as we could. Now, normally I hated taking pictures, because I loathed the way I looked in them. But, for this special occasion I would take plenty. So, I take a picture with two of my close friends, and when we look at the picture, I was horrified!

Could I be that big? This couldn't be true!!! I knew I was overweight, but when I saw myself in this picture it was an eye-opening experience. I did not want it posted on Facebook, Instagram, or anywhere else for that matter. But, I was too afraid to speak up and tell my friend to delete the awful picture!! So, of course it went all over the popular social networks…ugh!! That day, I decided this is not okay. I am the only one who can do something about this, and it was time to get busy. I decided I was going to take out my sew-in and get some braids (for me, braids represent it is time to get down and dirty with the workout plan). That picture ignited a flame of motivation in me. That motivation that I had been lacking was jumpstarted. I was ready. It was time to get to work.

My first step was to go to the doctor. I hated going to the doctor. Why? Because one of the first things they do is check your weight. I didn't want to see that! Well, once again, I was horrified. I was the biggest I had ever been in my life. Before my doctor's visit, I did a little research, and diagnosed myself with Thyroid disease. I had researched the signs, and while I had a majority of the symptoms, I didn't have them all. That wasn't important to me because the symptoms I did have was enough to convince me! In my eyes, I had it. It made sense. My father has it, and both of my grandmothers had it. While at the doctor's office, I shared with him what I researched, and he agreed that this could be a possibility. This gave me a little hope. He recommended that I follow up with my primary care physician just to make sure. No problem! I made the appointment with new hope that I had thyroid disease, and that it could be treated, and all this weight would go away. Boy was I wrong.

I pull up to the doctor's office ready to state my case and prove to him that I had this disease. Then, he would give me a magic pill that would cure it all. Yeah, right. I get in the office with my doctor and I start to present my evidence to support my self-diagnosis. I told him about the symptoms I'd been experiencing, which matched those of thyroid disease, and how several members of my family have it. Either he was not listening to me, or he was not buying it. He went on to tell me that he tested me a couple of years ago and I did not have it. I remember thinking just because I didn't have it then, does not mean I don't have it now!! I had gained forty pounds in less than three years! I didn't consume "juices and berries" all the time, but I didn't eat any more than anyone else, and I was fairly active. It just didn't make sense to me. Well, he looks at my weight and told me that it was a lot of weight. He asked me my height and I responded, "5'9"." He looked over a chart, and told me I was three pounds away from being morbidly obese. I remember that statement taking my breath away. Did I hear him correctly? Morbidly obese....who me? Then, the tears started to flow. Everything else he told me was a blur. When he stepped out of the office I called a good friend of mine crying my eyes out. She tried to encourage me, and even offered to come be with me. My doctor returned with some other heavy statements for me. He told me he was going to get me a battery of tests (thyroid, diabetes, cholesterol, and some others). He also had some possible options for me. One was to offer me a pill that would help curb my appetite. Another was to try *Weight Watchers*, or other programs like it. He even mentioned giving me a pill for depression that has a fifty-percent chance of helping with weight loss. If that didn't work, he stated that I may want to think about gastric by-pass surgery. What? A pill for depression? Who said I was depressed? Gastric by-pass surgery? My head was spinning! This made me cry even harder, and I couldn't take anymore. I had to get out of there. I was still in tears as I left and I just shut down. I didn't want to talk about it at all. I had shared my self-diagnosis with several people. I was embarrassed, and also at a loss as to what to do next. I remember my mom wanting to talk about it, and her telling me some things I could do differently. I remember saying, "Mommy, I don't want to talk about it". As she continued, I remember getting so angry and thinking to myself: "How many times do I have to say I don't want to talk about it?" I just did not want to talk or be around anybody. I was on a pity bus all by myself. Even after all of that, I was still holding on to hope that I had thyroid disease. How crazy is that? Who actually wishes for a disease? Yep, you guessed it. Me!

Well my wait was over. It had been a week and my test results were back. Everything came back negative. No diabetes, no high cholesterol, and most of all, no thyroid disease. What? You have got to be kidding me? I am in total disbelief. I called my doctor's receptionist to verify my counts again for my thyroid test, and she told me they were way in the safe zone. What do I do? I went into a full-blown outcry. Instead of being grateful that I did not have any of these conditions, I got upset. How ungrateful is that? I should have been screaming from the mountaintops, "Thank you, Jesus!" Instead, I got back on my pity bus, and refused to accept what was staring me right in the face. The problem with my weight was ME! Yes, the problem was me, myself, and I.

Finally, I decided to pick myself up and get busy. I was determined. The only one who could change my situation was me. I had run out of excuses and April 19, 2013 was the day that I changed my life for good.

While I was on this journey, I also learned so much about how I felt about myself. I reflected on being bullied as a child. Not physically, but verbally. I know we were brought up with the old saying, "Sticks and stones may break my bones, but words will never hurt me." To me, that is the biggest lie in history. I kept all of those hurt feelings inside. I never told anyone what I was going through. My bullies made fun of my clothes, my shoes, my hair, but most of all, my looks. I mean, some would come off as joking, but while they were joking, I was hurting by their words. I was a beautiful, chocolate girl, but I didn't realize it. I never felt pretty at all! I was always the cool one, but never the one that guys really wanted to date. I mean, don't get me wrong, I had boyfriends, but they were few and far between. This along with the bullying took a toll on my self-esteem. Until recently, I never knew how much it affected me. I always made sure that I never left the house until I was well put together. I would buy my clothes according to what I thought others would like. Once I started working at age 14, I made a vow to myself that this would not continue to happen. They stopped making fun of me about my clothes, but the damage was already done. Since I never dealt with those hurt feelings as a child, I carried those things over into adulthood. I also realized that I never looked at my face in the mirror. I know you are wondering, "How do you not look at your face in the mirror?" Easy! I would look everywhere else instead of looking at my face as a whole. How did I finally realize this? I am so glad you asked. I was at a gas station and I saw this guy I had a huge crush on. I knew I was dressed cute, so I was hoping he would notice me that day. Well, we sat there and talked for five minutes or so, and then we parted ways. I got back in my car and happened to glance in my rear view mirror, and to my horror, I noticed that I had white stuff all over my face! I was horrified! My mind was racing! I quickly began thinking and wondering if this was all over my face the entire time? After that incident, I started to notice that I never looked in the mirror while I was getting dressed. I would look at my hair, my neck, and lips, but never into my own eyes through the mirror. Why? The only thing I could come up with is that I never felt comfortable with who I saw in the mirror. To this day I have to constantly remember to look at myself in the mirror. I have to remind myself daily that I am pretty, and that I am good enough. Again, it is a process. I realized that this is only something I can change, and I will, one day at a time.

During my journey I have learned many things. I have lost weight before, but not like this. Not only have I lost weight, but I have gained knowledge. I have learned how to change my lifestyle, and not how to diet. I've learned to eliminate excuses. I am now honest with myself. I now know that this process is ninety-nine percent mental, and one percent physical. Most of all, I've learned how to love and be happy with me. It has been two years since I began my weight loss journey, and I would like to share it with you. As of today, I have lost over sixty pounds and counting. My journey has not been easy, but I made it, and so can you.

## Reflection on Chapter 1

- Do you feel you can relate to my journey in any way? If so, how?

___

___

___

- What excuses have you used before to explain your weight gain, or any other issue you struggle with?

___

___

___

Notes:

___

___

___

___

# Chapter 2

~Speak life, not defeat, into your situation. Know you can do it! ~

Monica McLaurine

## Believe in Yourself

Sometimes, we can defeat ourselves before we even get started. I don't have time to work out. "I can't do all of those exercises. I tried before, and I didn't lose any weight." These are just a few of the things we say to ourselves that keep us from working out. I have learned that we can be our own worst enemy. What we fail to realize is that the power of life and death is in the tongue. Stop speaking defeat into your situation. So many times I have heard people say they can't do this, or they don't have the time. Yes, you can, and yes, you do! Will it, or can it be challenging? Yes, it could be. You have a family, or two jobs, and you don't see where you can make time for it. Oh and here is my favorite: "eating healthy is too expensive". Look, I know you are busy. We all are.

You owe it to yourself to be healthy. That same family you are claiming takes up so much of your time needs you. It will take some sacrificing, but you can do it. I am not a fitness guru by any means, but I do know that weight loss mainly takes these two important components: controlling your diet and regular exercise. I am not saying that you have to work out three times a day, only eat celery and carrots, and drink nothing but water. You have to find out what will work best for you. I tried a few weight loss programs that worked for others, but they didn't work for me. There are an abundance of programs for weight management, and supplements that can assist you with your goals. I encourage you to research and try some of these programs. Then, you need to implement a workout plan. I am sorry, but there is no way around it. Be honest with yourself about your time. Can you find an extra twenty to thirty minutes before your family gets up and moving for the day? Can you go for a brisk walk on your lunch break? What about after your kids are off to bed and the house is quiet? Can you find a workout DVD, or cable workout program you can do before bed? Okay, you say you have very little willpower when it comes to your eating. Have you ever tried the online program/app *MyFitnessPal*? There are also several other programs out there that can help you keep up with your caloric intake, carbs, and other essential things you need to monitor while changing your diet. You need to become aware of the many options you have to assist you in living a healthy lifestyle. Many people have asked me, "What worked for you?" My answer, "I would just watch my caloric intake, with the assistance of *MyFitnessPal*, and exercising five days a week." Now, it is time to find out what works for YOU!

## The Power of Your Mind

Now, let's talk about the power of the mind. I have been an athlete of some sort pretty much all of my life. My problem was the lack of motivation to get up and do something about my weight. I would whine about how tired I was after working two jobs, and just lacked motivation. I had friends and family all around me who were taking control and maintaining their healthy lifestyles. That should have been my motivation and model. I mean, I had lost weight before, and I could do it again, couldn't I? This should have been all the motivation I needed, right? Wrong! I was not motivated at all. I would cheer them on, and go home. I knew I was overweight, but my mind was not in the right place. I was not mentally ready to change my lifestyle. I was always talking about how tired I was, and how I didn't have the energy. Telling myself this aloud, and in my thoughts, gave me the excuse not to go and workout. I should have been telling myself that I could muster up the strength to do it, and that I could manage my time better. There were so many things I could have been telling myself, instead of giving myself excuses. I had to learn to motivate myself and eliminate my excuses. I had to believe in myself and you have to do the same. I believe in you! Now believe in yourself.

Also make sure you surround yourself with like-minded people who will encourage you. Believe it or not, being surrounded by positive people can make a huge difference. Sometimes you will get tired, and feel complacent with day-to-day life, and you will need others to help push you. There were several times when I felt like giving up, and would have to call on people to speak life into me at that moment. Their words would give me that extra push to keep going. Sometimes, they would even pop-up without me asking. I can remember an instance when I convinced myself that it would be okay to skip a day one week instead of going my usual five. It really wouldn't hurt anything, right? I mean, I was going to the gym every week religiously, so taking this one day off would be okay, wouldn't it? Well, at that very moment, I went to check my inbox on Facebook and I had a message from a dear friend with a message encouraging me to keep doing what I was doing, and that I inspired him. I remember being wowed and thinking, "How did he know?" "Was he watching me the whole time?" I could not believe it! But, you know what? It was just what I needed to get up and go to the gym. I also had friends and acquaintances that were on the same journey as I was. We would call each other to whine and complain, but when it was all over and done with, we would go and workout. We would go through the same struggles and triumphs, so we could always relate to what the other person was going through. We could work through it together because we were on the same team. This type of support is most valuable and is much needed.

The majority of this journey is mental. The more you can speak life into yourself, and surround yourself with positive people, the better. Remember to believe in yourself. You can do it!

## Reflections Chapter 2

1. What are some of the reasons that keep your from choosing a healthier lifestyle?

______________________________________________

______________________________________________

______________________________________________

2. Do you sometimes allow negative thoughts and excuses to cause doubt in yourself? How does this affect your health and weight goals? Or any other goals you have?

______________________________________________

______________________________________________

______________________________________________

Notes:

______________________________________________

______________________________________________

______________________________________________

______________________________________________

# Chapter 3

~Just because it is hard, doesn't mean you can't do it. Believe in yourself. ~

Monica McLaurine

## What Is Your Plan?

In reaching my goals, I had to figure out how I was going to accomplish my healthy lifestyle. How much weight did I want to lose? What was it going to take to get it done? Did I want to try *Weight Watchers*, again? How many times would I have to exercise each week? How long would it take to accomplish my goals? Am I really ready to put all of my effort into losing this weight? Yes, these were all questions that were running through my head. I knew I needed to have a plan if I was going to be successful. I think that is why so many people struggle through this process. I mean, you are pumped and ready to go, but you are running yourself in circles. You see no quick results, so you get discouraged and quit. You have to start with a plan. This was

**Visit with your doctor**

There can be a variety of reasons why you may be having issues with your weight. Yes, it is obvious that you may be overeating, but you could also have some serious health issues. These could also hinder your progress. You could have several issues, including thyroid disease. Hypothyroidism, also called underactive **thyroid** disease, is a common disorder. With hypothyroidism your thyroid gland does not make enough thyroid hormone. The thyroid gland is located in the front lower part of your neck. Hormones released by the gland travel through your bloodstream and affect nearly every part of your body, from your **heart** and **brain**, to your muscles and **skin**. The thyroid controls how your body's cells use energy from food, a process called **metabolism**. Among other things, your metabolism affects your body's temperature, your heartbeat, and how well you burn calories. If you don't have enough thyroid hormone, your body processes slow down. That means your body makes less energy, and your metabolism becomes sluggish (WebMD, LLC., 2014). Common signs of an underactive thyroid are tiredness, weight gain, and depression. An underactive thyroid is not usually serious. It can often be treated successfully by taking daily hormone tablets to replace the hormones your thyroid isn't making (National Health Service, 2014). Remember, this is the medical condition that I convinced myself that I had. Fortunately, I did not.

There are some medications that can cause weight gain, Paxil, Prednisone, and several anti-depression medications, just to name a few. You also need to check with your doctor to make sure you can handle exercise and change in your diet. I don't mean to give you a lesson in medications or medical conditions. I just want you to make sure you have the "okay" from your doctor before you start you weight loss journey. You want to make sure your body is physically ready to take on this activity. I want you to get healthy, but do it in the right way.

**Choose the right fitness plan**

There are so many fitness and weight loss plans out now that it can be overwhelming sometimes. The most important thing is to pick the plan that is best for you (your doctor can also help with this). When I started, I tried *Weight Watchers* for three months. I didn't lose a pound. I know several people who have used this plan, and have been very successful. It just didn't work for me.

Another example is the *Body by Vi* shake and cereal plan. Oh boy! I can't count the people I know who either sell it, and/or have been successful at losing weight and keeping it off. This is a movement! Yet again, it didn't work for me.

I know you are thinking "What worked for you?" What works for me is working out four to five times a week, and watching my caloric intake. That may be the basis for every weight loss plan, but this plan works for me. When I first started I did one hour of cardio, five times a week. Then, I would work on my abs, arms, and legs on alternating days to complement my cardio workout. Some people would ask me why I did so much cardio, and my answer is simple, "I wanted to burn as many calories as possible". Now, there are several ways you can burn calories, but again this is what worked best for me. Also, when you are trying to pick a plan, don't be afraid to ask for advice. One thing I have found is that more and more people are striving to live healthy. No, everyone is not an expert, or an exercise guru, but they can give you some insight on what worked for them. You never know, they could have some of the same issues you are dealing with, and give you good information that could help you.

**Get your mind right!**

Get in your mental zone. Talk to yourself. Encourage yourself. You have to plan how many days a week you want to work out. To lose weight, I feel you need four to five days of exercise a week. I know, I know. That sounds like a lot! You have to put in the work. You mentally prepare yourself to do it. Remember, you want to be healthy, and this is a big part in getting there. Pack your gym bag the night if possible, I know I am always rushing. You don't want to chance forgetting something that may prevent you from working out. I was notorious for trying to pack my gym bag in the morning, and forgetting something. I would sometimes forget my gym shoes, my workout shirt, workout pants, and even my socks! At one point in time it was a running joke with a guy at the gym on, "What did I forget today?" Some days I would be so confident that I had everything, and I would go back to the locker room to find out that was not the case. We'd both get a big laugh out of that.

If you work out at home, set a time you are going to work out and stick to it. I know there will be times when you may have to adjust this, but it is very important to keep a schedule. Put it in your appointment calendar. Your workout should be just as important as any other appointment you may have. You owe it to yourself.

Another thing I found that helped me is packing my lunch. I am sure you know that eating out every day can be expensive. Also, know that eating healthy, and eating out every day, can be very expensive (at least for me). Grocery shopping and pre-packaging saves me a lot of time and money. You have everything you need for the day and it cuts cost dramatically.

In addition to cutting cost, packing your meals will help you control your portions and calorie intake. When you pack your meals at night, you can put your meals and snacks in the correct portions. Once your meal and/or snack are gone, they are gone. I know I am not the only one who goes back and grabs another portion or snack when I am at home, or am I? Well, I've been guilty of that many times. If you package your lunch and snacks, there is no more to go back and get. If you have a problem with controlling your portions, this will definitely help you. You may be thinking it may be hard to do, but trust me, it's not. It usually takes a few weeks to form a habit, so start making this a habit! You can do it!

## Reflection Chapter 3

1. Have you discussed your fitness goals with your doctor? What recommendations did your doctor have for you?

2. What is your plan of action for a healthier lifestyle?

Notes:

# *Chapter 4*

## Hope is needed. Don't let past failures kill your hope.

Monica McLaurine

**Find ways to hold yourself accountable**

Keeping yourself accountable is a major key to your success. It is easy to get distracted and frustrated during your journey. During these times you need to figure out little ways to keep yourself motivated. These are a few of the accountability triggers that worked for me:

**Share your journey**

I remember when I first started my journey I didn't want to share it. I was embarrassed. I had come to the realization that I had really let myself go. I mean, who wants to admit that publicly? Not me! Well, I remember one Sunday morning as I sat in church, God spoke to me and told me I needed to share what I had been going through. Boy, am I glad I was obedient. The day after losing my first twenty-four pounds, I decided to share my story on Facebook. I never imagined the response would be so great. I received so many likes, posts, and inbox messages from so many people. They came from friends, family, and even people I didn't know. They were so supportive, it brought me to tears. Not only were there supportive posts and messages, there were also people who were in the same boat as I was. They asked what was I doing to lose the weight, and they were asking what they could do to start on their own journeys. I was floored. My journey was not just for me, it was to help and encourage others as well. I realize that now, and gladly accept the challenge.

You may ask, "How this will hold you accountable?" Well, people are watching you now. Some will be supportive, and some will not. Some you will inspire and others will secretly think you won't accomplish your goal and keep it off. Either way, if you are like me, both are motivation. If you support me, and you are inspired by my journey, I am going to do whatever it takes to continue to inspire you. There were many whose stories inspired me to keep going. I will continue to share my story to help others and it is my honor to do so. Now to the naysayers, I can show you better than I can tell you. Watch me work!!

## Get rid of your old stuff

A few years back I lost a total of fifty pounds. I remember being so proud of myself. A good friend of mine congratulated me, and told me to get rid of my old clothes because I was not going back. I remember saying, "I can't do that! I may need them in case I gain my weight back." I remember him saying, "Okay, you need to get rid of those clothes." At that time, I did not realize how my words would come back to haunt me. I kept all of those clothes. So, when I regained my weight (and then some) ~~back~~, I always had something in my closet that fit. It was a smooth transition for me to gain all of my weight back. I made it easy for myself. I should have taken my friend's advice.

This time I remembered that advice. If it is too big, and does not look good on me, it's taking up space and has to go. This serves as a trigger for me. If it is getting too tight, I know I need to tighten up and get back on task. Also, I had to get rid of some of my shoes as well. Although it was very traumatic for me to get rid of my shoes (shoe lovers will feel me on this), I know I am not going back, so I would not be able to wear them anymore anyway. So why not give them to someone who can use them? The last time I made it easy for myself to regain the weight. Not this time. I am getting rid of it all. This has also given me the opportunity to be a blessing to others. I am not bragging or anything, but I had some nice clothes and shoes, and I wanted to give them to someone who needed/wanted them. Once there was a friend of mine who I gave a lot of clothes and shoes. She told me that she concentrated so much on getting things for her kids, that she was not able to do anything for herself. I was so humbled to be able to assist her. We can get so caught up in ourselves that we can forget to be a blessing to others.

**Get an accountability partner**

An accountability partner is crucial for your journey. It is always helpful if this person is on the same path as you are. To me there is a fine line between motivating someone, and being hurtful to someone who is trying to lose weight. Most are just trying to be helpful, but sometimes the comments that are meant to help can tear a person down. The wrong statement could cause someone to backslide. So make sure your accountability partner is someone who is positive, and believes in you. They will push you to keep going when you feel like giving up. They will work out with you, and encourage you along the way. They also won't beat you up if you slack off a little. They will speak life into you and help give you that little extra spark you need to go that extra mile. You also need to give them the same motivation in return. You can celebrate each other's goals and snap each other into shape when you fall off. Trust me, during your journey you will need that.

Often times, when you're only accountable to yourself, it's easy to become lax. If you and your partner are scheduled to go for a quick run every Monday and Wednesday, and you choose not to go, you're not only letting yourself down, but your partner as well. You are counting on each other, and you don't want to let that other person down. You could also be giving your partner an excuse not to exercise because they may not want to work out alone. Don't give them an excuse!! They are counting on you! Don't let them down!

## Reflection Chapter 4

1. In what ways are you keeping yourself accountable?

_______________________________________________

_______________________________________________

_______________________________________________

3. Name two people that you'd pick as your accountability/workout partners. Why?

_______________________________________________

_______________________________________________

_______________________________________________

Notes:

_______________________________________________

_______________________________________________

_______________________________________________

_______________________________________________

# *Chapter 5*

## ~Refuse to quit! You owe it to yourself! ~

Monica McLaurine

## Document your journey

### Say cheese!

Documenting your journey is essential. When losing weight it can be hard sometimes to see, or feel a change in your body. I weighed myself once a week at the beginning of my journey. I was happy to see the weight coming off on the scale, but I could not see it in the mirror. It actually took for me to lose thirty pounds before I could see the weight loss without having to look at pictures. I captured my weight through pictures in ten pound increments. Doing this really helped a lot. It helped me stay focused. I still go back to those pictures often to remind myself of how far I have come on my journey. It still amazes me. I remember taking those pictures and being so proud of myself. I was really doing it this time, and the pictures really kept me on track.

## <u>Blog about it</u>

I think it is important to keep some type of journal of your journey. Some people are very private about their journey, while others, like me, are more vocal. When I would speak to people about my struggles and funny moments during this journey it was suggested to me that I should blog about it. I remember thinking, "Yeah, right! I don't know anything about blogging." Boy, am I glad I started blogging. I actually enjoy it. Not only have I gotten favorable responses from others, it has also been therapeutic and encouraging to me. I try to keep them short and sweet, but informative for all that view it. There are plenty of free sites you can use. So give it a try. You just might like it.

**Keep a written journal**

I know that some of you all are not into the whole internet-online thing. That's okay, but you still need to document your journey. Invest in a journal where you can keep up with your progress. I used to think that this process was useless, but I was wrong. This is another way to keep yourself accountable. So many times I found myself, and several other people have often wondered what we have done to pack on these extra pounds. Once I started to write down what I was eating daily, I began to understand where those pounds were coming from. Sometimes we think we are eating healthier, when we're really not. Let me give you an example. You love salads with all of the vegetables you can stand on them. Then, you top it off with ranch, or blue cheese salad dressing. Or, you give yourself a food cheat day that turns into an entire weekend of cheating. The next thing you know, five or more pounds have crept back on.

When you document what you are eating and drinking every day, it helps you see for yourself what you are doing wrong. It is hard to dispute your counter-productive eating habits when it written down right in front of your face.

## Reflections Chapter 5

1. In what ways do you plan to document your journey?

______________________________________________

______________________________________________

______________________________________________

2. What measures did you use previously to keep yourself accountable?

______________________________________________

______________________________________________

______________________________________________

Notes:

______________________________________________

______________________________________________

______________________________________________

______________________________________________

# Chapter 6

~Don't be afraid to ask for help. Everyone needs help sometimes. Don't let your pride keep you from succeeding! ~

Monica McLaurine

## Getting rid of your internal junk

Many times people walk around as if everything is

cream", like they have never had a bad day. Truth be told, a lot of us have internal issues we really need to deal with. We just don't realize how much that internal junk affects us. Because of my internal junk, one of the things I realized, as I pointed out earlier, was that I didn't look at my face in the mirror. I carried around a lot of unwanted and unneeded baggage that affected the way I felt about myself.

We have to realize that these issues will not go away by themselves. We have to deal with them. This is something I had to learn along the way. Dealing with these issues wasn't always easy, but I had to deal with them in order to become whole. These are some of the things I have dealt with, and how I am tackling my internal junk.

## Dealing with the person in the mirror

Over the years, I acquired a few insecurities about myself. I never felt happy with myself. I felt I was never good enough. No matter how well I dressed, or what pair of sexy shoes I wore, I still felt deficient. I was that girl whose boyfriends were very few and far between, and I never understood why. All around me friends and family were dating, getting married, and having families. Then you had me, the one who was always in a dead-end relationship. This weighed on me heavily. Again, I thought, "What is wrong with me?" These were questions I asked myself over and over again. After a while, it really affected the way I felt about myself. Even though I desired to have a mate, I was starting to believe that it was never going to happen. Slowly I began to love the person I saw in the mirror and not constantly wonder what was wrong with me. I started to look for the good things about myself and not always at the things that were wrong. I couldn't expect others to see the inside and outer beauty I possessed and not see those qualities myself. I changed my mindset and I finally love my own reflection.

**Bullying effects are stronger than you think**

Throughout elementary and middle school I was bullied. No one ever physically attacked me, but they did so emotionally. All bullying is terrible, but emotional bullying, to me, is one of the worst types. I was teased about not having the type of clothes everyone else was wearing. I was also made fun of because I was dark-skinned. The hurtful things that were said to me still resonate with me to this very day. We can say all day that they're just words, and they can't hurt you. That is the biggest lie in history. They do hurt! Those words that were said to me, so many years ago, still stay with me.

Also, more times than not, the clothes I bought were not bought because I liked them. I bought clothes that I thought others would like. The shoes I bought, most of the time, were also for this same reason. Remember, I was picked on because I didn't have all the clothes that everyone else was wearing. Because of that, I stood out amongst everyone else. They would have a field day embarrassing me in from of other kids. I would grin and bear it, like it was all a big joke.

All of that teasing I endured was in my head. I felt like I had something to prove to others. I never shared what was going on with me, so I never had the chance to get reassurance that it didn't matter what others thought of me. I took it all in stride (so I thought), and acted as if nothing was wrong. All along, I was secretly dying inside from the after effects of my past bullying episodes.

## Don't be afraid to grab some couch

Throughout the years, I carried this baggage with me. I carried it for so long I didn't even realize I was still holding on to it. Once I realized what I was doing to myself, I finally decided that I had to deal with it. You cannot change what you don't acknowledge. I could no longer deal with all of this bottled up hurt and anger.

When I was going through my weight loss journey, I had to ask myself some hard questions. This was not an easy task, but a needed one. While I was making progress dealing with my issues, I realized I needed some additional help. I decided to seek out a therapist. I know sometimes when someone admits to seeing a therapist they can get the side eye from others, but this was one of the best decisions I have ever made.

Some say that they don't want to open up to a complete stranger, and tell them all of their business. Well, that is exactly why I was in favor of going to therapy. I wanted someone who didn't know me. I didn't want to worry about being judged by confiding in someone I already knew. I needed someone who could be objective with no pre-conceived notions about me. A person who could remain neutral, and can see things that were buried deep down inside my soul. That is what therapy did for me.

In the beginning, I found myself holding back. I was not telling her what I really needed to deal with. I had to let down my security wall for a chance to really uncover some things that were holding me back. I have to admit that at first I was very uncomfortable. I remember after my initial appointment feeling so heavy with emotion that I wondered if I was doing the right thing. Well, I was. She helped me to see things clearly, and continue progressing on my journey. She helped me to open up, and expose my issues that I had been hiding behind my beautiful smile. Once I opened up, and trusted the process, I was on my way to healing. I had so many things deeply buried that I had forgotten about them. It was at that point that I realized what I mentioned earlier, "You can't change things you won't acknowledge." I was determined to change, and if this is what I needed to do, I was going to do it.

My therapy sessions were life-changing. I recommend that everyone spend some time on a therapist couch. You may not have some of the same internal junk as me, but we all are dealing with something. Don't get caught up in stereotypes, and thinking therapy will not help you, because it will. Trust me. My therapist was there to help me, not to judge me and tell me what to do. She helped me think clearly about the direction I was going in. This was the help I needed, and wanted. I will continue to go in the future. Remember, this is a process, stick with it.

You may be wondering why I am sharing all of this. I am sharing this because we don't always realize how the baggage we carry around affects us. It can be toxic, and cause problems mentally, emotionally, and physically. I was dealing with my issues on my own, and unwavering in my quest to become better. This was, and will continue, to be a part of my process.

## Reflections Chapter 6

1. What are some of the unresolved issues you have?

______________________________________________

______________________________________________

______________________________________________

2. Would you be willing to try therapy? Do you believe it is a stigma in your community if you were to go to therapy? Why or why not?

______________________________________________

______________________________________________

______________________________________________

Notes:

______________________________________________

______________________________________________

______________________________________________

______________________________________________

# Chapter 7

~We all get frustrated sometimes. Don't get stuck in frustration, keep going! ~

Monica McLaurine

## The scale is not always your friend

When I began my journey, I weighed myself religiously every week. For the most part, my weight loss was consistent. I would have a setback here or there, but I always kept exercising. I weighed myself two to three times a week, and consistently saw weight loss. Then there came a time when I was continuing my workout routine, and not one pound was coming off of the scale. Now, I know about plateaus that you can experience when you lose weight. The plateaus are necessary, but so frustrating.

Just in case you are unfamiliar with what a weight-loss plateau is, let me explain it to you as my doctor explained it to me. After you start losing weight, your body needs time to adjust to the weight loss. During this adjustment is when you are most likely to experience a plateau. Don't get discouraged during this time. There are all types of information on how to break plateaus, but just know you have to go through it. Keep working out because it will pass. Stay in the fight!

**Your workout is like Groundhog Day**

Sometimes we get too comfortable with our workouts. We do the same workouts day in and day out. Though we continue to get a great workout, with plenty of sweat, what we do not realize is that our bodies can become used to our regime. When this happens, our workout regime may not be as effective as it was before.

Just like anything else, when we get comfortable we can occasionally become lax in our efforts. You may grow to become complacent with your workout, and may not put forth the same intensity as before. You have to switch up your routines. I have learned to vary my workout in order to trick my body. One day, I would do gym time with cardio, abs, and some arm work. Another day, I may go to an outdoor track, take a Zumba class, or tackle a staircase for some extreme cardio. These are just a few of my various workouts. Find ways to mix it up. You have to shock your body sometimes so it doesn't become stagnant. Don't be afraid to try new things. Have fun, try something new. You never know, you may find a new favorite workout!

## Sometimes life gets in the way

I know we all get busy sometimes, and it can affect our weight loss journeys. That's okay. Don't let this frustrate you. Keep your goal in sight. So what if you get caught up, and you miss a week, or two of working out, and you're eating everything. You have already made up in your mind that you are going to live healthier, and stay on your journey. Keep your promise to yourself. Get back in the gym, and get your eating back on track. You owe it to yourself. Do not let life make you lose focus. You did it before, so get back to it!

**Your weight can be very inconsistent**

This is something that always happens to me. My weight constantly fluctuates. I had to realize that I can't make a healthier lifestyle something I do every now and then. I finally realized that I had to be completely dedicated for this to work, and so do you. I continue to surround myself with positive people, and those who are on a similar path. Having like-minded people around me has been crucial to my journey. To be honest, I don't know what I would do without them. They constantly inspire me, and help me stay focused when my weight gets out of whack. They help ignite the spark that keeps me motivated. Thank you, guys!!

## Reflections Chapter 7

1. How often are you weighing yourself?

______________________________________________

______________________________________________

______________________________________________

2. How often are you switching up your workout? Are there any new workouts that you want to try?

______________________________________________

______________________________________________

______________________________________________

Notes:

______________________________________________

______________________________________________

______________________________________________

______________________________________________

# *Chapter 8*

~Moving on is not about forgetting, but learning from it, and becoming a stronger person. ~

Monica McLaurine

## What I've learned so Far

While going through my journey, my schedule was very busy. I worked two jobs (six days a week) and worked out five times a week. This gave me time to really examine myself from the inside out. I learned several things during this process and I hope these things will be beneficial to others on their journeys.

## I had to take control of my own self-esteem

If you have not done this, please do this as soon as possible. It is easy to blame others for our issues that may cause our low self-esteem. This process must begin and end with us.

I realized that I had to stop giving others so much power to affect my self-esteem. Yes, there were people and situations that may have contributed to my lack of self-esteem, but ultimately, I am the one who controls it. I had to really reach down deep to see where my self-esteem problem stemmed from. It stemmed mostly from experiences during in middle and high school years. I allowed these self-esteem issues to follow me into adulthood. I let what others said, or felt about me, affect how I looked at myself. Never again will I allow this to happen. Finally, I am now comfortable in my own skin. I finally love Monica! I am not saying that I am not receptive to constructive criticism, or unwilling to receive information that will help me. However, I am saying I will no longer allow others to have that much influence over me. If no one on this earth loves me, I love me. I am responsible for my own self-esteem. My journey was, and is so much more than weight loss. My journey was designed for me to finally learn how to love myself. It was for me to finally become comfortable in my own skin.

## Fat-shaming Does Not Help

As I stated before, I have had some people say some very hurtful things about my weight. A few of them claimed it was to help motivate me to do something about it. Guess what….that never helped me. If anything, it did more damage. Fat-shaming, or so called "tough love", can be counter-productive and very hurtful. Most people are already self-conscious, and unhappy, about their weight, and negative criticism does not help. I began my journey, not because of them, but because I was ready for a change. I made the decision of my own. No one else can make that decision for me.

I would also like to inspire others to know that if I can do it, so can they. So, instead of saying "You need to go to the gym!" maybe say, "Hey, I am going for a walk, would you like to join me?" Sometimes, it is not what you say, but how you say it. Then, if all else fails, back off a little. When they are ready, they will do it. Keep encouraging them.

**I would rather show them than tell them.**

I remember one day I received an inbox message from one of my constant supporters. The message I received went something like this, "I'm not meddling, but your second biggest challenge is for your haters. They are going to watch you like a hawk. Please do better than me and keep the weight off. Set a small gain weight of like five pounds, and never go over that five pound weight gain. It's awful when people can't celebrate with you. Love you!" This made me smile. One of the reasons is because it's nice to know that I have some die-hard supporters. The other reason was for my haters. I remember telling her that I knew I had haters out there, but that was okay because I needed them. They motivate me. People talked about me before my weight loss, and they are talking about me now. Rather than strike back at them, or lose my focus worrying about them, I decided I would show them better than I could tell them. This healthier lifestyle I chose to embark on is about me, and no one else. I have nothing to prove to anyone.

So, I say all of that to say, "Let people talk about you. Don't get mad about it, use it!" You can find motivation from anywhere, so add this one to your list. Give them something to really talk about. Who knows, you may even motivate them to live healthier.

**Motivation is part of my calling**

When I started my journey, I had no idea about what God had in store for me. I remember when I lost my first twenty-four pounds I heard God clearly tell me to share my journey. At first, I was ashamed, but then I decided to be obedient. My goodness, I had no idea that transparency about my journey would touch so many lives. From that day forward, I began to receive numerous phone calls, text and inbox messages of encouragement, and requests for my advice. I was literally blown away. I had no idea that my journey could inspire others. This is when I discovered my journey was not just about me. It was also for me to influence others to start their own journeys and that is what I will continue to do with humbleness and honor.

## Reflections Chapter 8

1. Have you ever experienced fat-shaming? If so, how did it make you feel?

______________________________________________

______________________________________________

______________________________________________

2. Do you have low self-esteem?

______________________________________________

______________________________________________

______________________________________________

3. Name some of the most important things you learned about yourself from reading this book.

______________________________________________

______________________________________________

______________________________________________

Notes:

______________________________________________

______________________________________________

______________________________________________

______________________________________________

# Chapter 9

~"A great habit for self-growth is routinely making and breaking habits."~

-Colin Wright

# Creating New Habits

It has been said that it can take anywhere from twenty-one to thirty days to create a new habit. For those who are starting their journeys to a healthier lifestyle, or whatever goals you set for your life, I have found that journaling really helps with this process. Some people prefer to use electronic journals, such as *MyFitnessPal,* while others prefer to use pen and paper.

I just don't want this book to be a one-time read. I want you to refer back for motivation, and as a place for you to record your journey. So, I have included a daily journal for you to use to get started. In your journal, keep up with your caloric intake, exercise, progress, and any information you deem pertinent for you. Also, please do not put too much emphasis on your weight loss for the first month. The weight loss will come. Stay focused on your journey, stay consistent and the rest will come.

Note: This may be an adjustment for some, but hang in there. It will be worth it. Trust me on this. Happy journaling!

# Creating New Habits

## Starting Measurements

Then the LORD said to me,

"Write my answer plainly on tablets,
so that a runner can carry the correct message to others"
Habakkuk 2:2

Starting Weight: ______________

Goal Weight: _________________

Exercise Per Week Goal: ________________

Caloric In-take Per Day Goal: ____________

Daily Water In-take Goal: _______________

Other personal goals:

__________________________________________________________

__________________________________________________________

__________________________________________________________

__________________________________________________________

# Weekly Motivation

# Week One:

## Starting New

"Don't bring the bricks from your past into the present. If you are not careful, you will end up building the same house. Let the past go!" - Wess Morgan

## **Day One:**

Daily Exercise: ______________________________

Calories Burned: ______________________________

Daily Caloric Intake: _________________________

Water Intake: _______________________

Daily Reflections:

_______________________________________________________

_______________________________________________________

_______________________________________________________

_______________________________________________________

_______________________________________________________

# Weekly Motivation

## Week One:

Starting Anew

"Don't bring the bricks from your past into the present. If you are not careful, you will end up building the same house. Let the past go!" - Wess Morgan

## Day Two:

Daily Exercise: ______________________________

Calories Burned: ______________________________

Daily Caloric Intake: __________________________

Water Intake: _______________________

Daily Reflections:

________________________________________________________

________________________________________________________

________________________________________________________

________________________________________________________

________________________________________________________

# Weekly Motivation

## Week One:

### Starting Anew

"Don't bring the bricks from your past into the present. If you are not careful, you will end up building the same house. Let the past go!" - Wess Morgan

## **Day Three:**

Daily Exercise: ______________________________

Calories Burned: ______________________________

Daily Caloric Intake: __________________________

Water Intake: _______________________

Daily Reflections:

________________________________________________________

________________________________________________________

________________________________________________________

________________________________________________________

# Weekly Motivation

## Week One:

Starting Anew

"Don't bring the bricks from your past into the present. If you are not careful, you will end up building the same house. Let the past go!" -Wess Morgan

## **Day Four:**

Daily Exercise: ______________________________

Calories Burned: ____________________________

Daily Caloric Intake: _________________________

Water Intake: ______________________

Daily Reflections:

_______________________________________________________

_______________________________________________________

_______________________________________________________

_______________________________________________________

_______________________________________________________

# Weekly Motivation

## Week One:

### Starting Anew

"Don't bring the bricks from your past into the present. If you are not careful, you will end up building the same house. Let the past go!" -Wess Morgan

## **Day Five:**

Daily Exercise: ______________________________

Calories Burned: _____________________________

Daily Caloric Intake: _________________________

Water Intake: _______________________

Daily Reflections:

_______________________________________________________

_______________________________________________________

_______________________________________________________

_______________________________________________________

_______________________________________________________

# Weekly Motivation

## Week One:

### Starting Anew

"Don't bring the bricks from your past into the present. If you are not careful, you will end up building the same house. Let the past go!" -Wess Morgan

## **Day Six:**

Daily Exercise: ______________________________

Calories Burned: ____________________________

Daily Caloric Intake: _________________________

Water Intake: _______________________

Daily Reflections:

_______________________________________________________

_______________________________________________________

_______________________________________________________

_______________________________________________________

_______________________________________________________

# Weekly Motivation

## Week One:

### Starting Anew

"Don't bring the bricks from your past into the present. If you are not careful, you will end up building the same house. Let the past go!" -Wess Morgan

## Day Seven:

Daily Exercise: ______________________________

Calories Burned: ____________________________

Daily Caloric Intake: _________________________

Water Intake: ______________________

Daily Reflections:

______________________________________________________

______________________________________________________

______________________________________________________

______________________________________________________

______________________________________________________

# Weekly Motivation

## Week Two:

The Company You Keep

Surround yourself with like-minded people. Find others who have the similar goals so you can encourage each other.

## Day Eight:

Daily Exercise: ______________________________

Calories Burned: ______________________________

Daily Caloric Intake: __________________________

Water Intake: ______________________

Daily Reflections:

________________________________________________________

________________________________________________________

________________________________________________________

________________________________________________________

# Weekly Motivation

## Week Two:

### The Company You Keep

Surround yourself with like-minded people. Find others who have the similar goals so you can encourage each other.

### Day Nine:

Daily Exercise: ______________________________

Calories Burned: _____________________________

Daily Caloric Intake: __________________________

Water Intake: _______________________

Daily Reflections:

_______________________________________________________

_______________________________________________________

_______________________________________________________

_______________________________________________________

_______________________________________________________

# Weekly Motivation

## Week Two:

### The Company You Keep

Surround yourself with like-minded people. Find others who have the similar goals so you can encourage each other.

## Day Ten:

Daily Exercise: ______________________________

Calories Burned: ____________________________

Daily Caloric Intake: _________________________

Water Intake: _______________________

Daily Reflections:

_______________________________________________________

_______________________________________________________

_______________________________________________________

_______________________________________________________

_______________________________________________________

# Weekly Motivation

## Week Two:

### The Company You Keep

Surround yourself with like-minded people. Find others who have the similar goals so you can encourage each other.

## Day Eleven:

Daily Exercise: ______________________________

Calories Burned: ____________________________

Daily Caloric Intake: _________________________

Water Intake: ______________________

Daily Reflections:

_______________________________________________________

_______________________________________________________

_______________________________________________________

_______________________________________________________

# Weekly Motivation

## Week Two:

### The Company You Keep

Surround yourself with like-minded people. Find others who have the similar goals so you can encourage each other.

## Day Twelve:

Daily Exercise: ______________________________

Calories Burned: ____________________________

Daily Caloric Intake: _________________________

Water Intake: _______________________

Daily Reflections:

________________________________________________________

________________________________________________________

________________________________________________________

________________________________________________________

# Weekly Motivation

## Week Two:

### The Company You Keep

Surround yourself with like-minded people. Find others who have the similar goals so you can encourage each other.

## Day Thirteen:

Daily Exercise: ______________________________

Calories Burned: ____________________________

Daily Caloric Intake: _________________________

Water Intake: ______________________

Daily Reflections:

________________________________________________________

________________________________________________________

________________________________________________________

________________________________________________________

# Weekly Motivation

## Week Two:

### The Company You Keep

Surround yourself with like-minded people. Find others who have the similar goals so you can encourage each other.

### Day Fourteen:

Daily Exercise: ______________________________

Calories Burned: ______________________________

Daily Caloric Intake: __________________________

Water Intake: ______________________

Daily Reflections:

_______________________________________________________

_______________________________________________________

_______________________________________________________

_______________________________________________________

# Weekly Motivation

## Week Three:

### Keep Your Focus

"Whenever you want to achieve something, keep your eyes open, concentrate and make sure you know exactly what it is you want. No one can hit their target with their eyes closed." -Paulo Coelho

## Day Fifteen:

Daily Exercise: ______________________________

Calories Burned: ______________________________

Daily Caloric Intake: __________________________

Water Intake: _______________________

Daily Reflections:

________________________________________________________

________________________________________________________

________________________________________________________

________________________________________________________

# Weekly Motivation

## Week Three:

### Keep Your Focus

"Whenever you want to achieve something, keep your eyes open, concentrate and make sure you know exactly what it is you want. No one can hit their target with their eyes closed." -Paulo Coelho

## Day Sixteen:

Daily Exercise: ______________________________

Calories Burned: ____________________________

Daily Caloric Intake: _________________________

Water Intake: _______________________

Daily Reflections:

________________________________________________________

________________________________________________________

________________________________________________________

________________________________________________________

# Weekly Motivation

## Week Three:

### Keep Your Focus

"Whenever you want to achieve something, keep your eyes open, concentrate and make sure you know exactly what it is you want. No one can hit their target with their eyes closed." -Paulo Coelho

## Day Seventeen:

Daily Exercise: ______________________________

Calories Burned: _____________________________

Daily Caloric Intake: _________________________

Water Intake: ______________________

Daily Reflections:

_______________________________________________________

_______________________________________________________

_______________________________________________________

_______________________________________________________

# Weekly Motivation

## Week Three:

### The Company You Keep

### Keep Your Focus

"Whenever you want to achieve something, keep your eyes open, concentrate and make sure you know exactly what it is you want. No one can hit their target with their eyes closed." -Paulo Coelho

## Day Eighteen:

Daily Exercise: ______________________________

Calories Burned: ______________________________

Daily Caloric Intake: __________________________

Water Intake: _______________________

Daily Reflections:

________________________________________________________

________________________________________________________

________________________________________________________

________________________________________________________

________________________________________________________

# Weekly Motivation

# Week Three:

## The Company You Keep

## Keep Your Focus

"Whenever you want to achieve something, keep your eyes open, concentrate and make sure you know exactly what it is you want. No one can hit their target with their eyes closed." -Paulo Coelho

## Day Nineteen:

Daily Exercise: ____________________________

Calories Burned: ___________________________

Daily Caloric Intake: _______________________

Water Intake: _____________________

Daily Reflections:

__________________________________________________

__________________________________________________

__________________________________________________

__________________________________________________

__________________________________________________

# Weekly Motivation

# Week Three:

**Keep Your Focus**

"Whenever you want to achieve something, keep your eyes open, concentrate and make sure you know exactly what it is you want. No one can hit their target with their eyes closed." -Paulo Coelho

## Day Twenty:

Daily Exercise: ______________________________

Calories Burned: _____________________________

Daily Caloric Intake: _________________________

Water Intake: _______________________

Daily Reflections:

________________________________________________________

________________________________________________________

________________________________________________________

________________________________________________________

________________________________________________________

# Weekly Motivation

# Week Three:

**Keep Your Focus**

"Whenever you want to achieve something, keep your eyes open, concentrate and make sure you know exactly what it is you want. No one can hit their target with their eyes closed." -Paulo Coelho

## Day Twenty-One:

Daily Exercise: ______________________________

Calories Burned: _____________________________

Daily Caloric Intake: _________________________

Water Intake: ______________________

Daily Reflections:

_______________________________________________________

_______________________________________________________

_______________________________________________________

_______________________________________________________

_______________________________________________________

# Weekly Motivation

# Week Three:

## Keep Your Focus

"Whenever you want to achieve something, keep your eyes open, concentrate and make sure you know exactly what it is you want. No one can hit their target with their eyes closed." -Paulo Coelho

## Day Twenty-Two:

Daily Exercise: ______________________________

Calories Burned: ____________________________

Daily Caloric Intake: _________________________

Water Intake: ______________________

Daily Reflections:

______________________________________________________

______________________________________________________

______________________________________________________

______________________________________________________

______________________________________________________

______________________________________________________

______________________________________________________

# Weekly Motivation

## Week Four:

"Persistence is the key

Many of life's failures are people who didn't realize how close they were to success when they gave up."

-Thomas Edison

## Day Twenty-Three:

Daily Exercise: ______________________________

Calories Burned: ____________________________

Daily Caloric Intake: _________________________

Water Intake: _______________________

Daily Reflections:

______________________________________________________

______________________________________________________

______________________________________________________

______________________________________________________

______________________________________________________

______________________________________________________

______________________________________________________

# Weekly Motivation

## Week Four:

"Persistence is the key

Many of life's failures are people who didn't realize how close they were to success when they gave up."

-Thomas Edison

## **Day Twenty-Four:**

Daily Exercise: ______________________________

Calories Burned: ______________________________

Daily Caloric Intake: __________________________

Water Intake: _______________________

Daily Reflections:

________________________________________________________

________________________________________________________

________________________________________________________

________________________________________________________

________________________________________________________

________________________________________________________

________________________________________________________

# Weekly Motivation

## Week Four:

"Persistence is the key

Many of life's failures are people who didn't realize how close they were to success when they gave up."

-Thomas Edison

## **Day Twenty-Five:**

Daily Exercise: ___________________________

Calories Burned: __________________________

Daily Caloric Intake: ______________________

Water Intake: ____________________

Daily Reflections:

_________________________________________________

_________________________________________________

_________________________________________________

_________________________________________________

_________________________________________________

_________________________________________________

_________________________________________________

# Weekly Motivation

## Week Four:

### Keep Your Focus

"Persistence is the key

Many of life's failures are people who didn't realize how close they were to success when they gave up."

-Thomas Edison

## Day Twenty-Six:

Daily Exercise: ______________________________

Calories Burned: _____________________________

Daily Caloric Intake: _________________________

Water Intake: _______________________

Daily Reflections:

________________________________________________________

________________________________________________________

________________________________________________________

________________________________________________________

________________________________________________________

________________________________________________________

# Weekly Motivation

# Week Four:

## Keep Your Focus

"Persistence is the key

Many of life's failures are people who didn't realize how close they were to success when they gave up."

-Thomas Edison

## Day Twenty-Seven:

Daily Exercise: ______________________________

Calories Burned: ______________________________

Daily Caloric Intake: __________________________

Water Intake: ______________________

Daily Reflections:

_______________________________________________________

_______________________________________________________

_______________________________________________________

_______________________________________________________

_______________________________________________________

_______________________________________________________

_______________________________________________________

# Weekly Motivation

## Week Four:

### Keep Your Focus

"Persistence is the key

Many of life's failures are people who didn't realize how close they were to success when they gave up."

-Thomas Edison

## Day Twenty-Eight:

Daily Exercise: ______________________________

Calories Burned: ____________________________

Daily Caloric Intake: _________________________

Water Intake: _______________________

Daily Reflections:

______________________________________________________

______________________________________________________

______________________________________________________

______________________________________________________

______________________________________________________

______________________________________________________

______________________________________________________

# Weekly Motivation

## Week Four:

**Keep Your Focus**

"Persistence is the key

Many of life's failures are people who didn't realize how close they were to success when they gave up."

-Thomas Edison

## Day Twenty-Nine:

Daily Exercise: ______________________________

Calories Burned: ____________________________

Daily Caloric Intake: _________________________

Water Intake: _______________________

*Daily Reflections:*

_______________________________________________________

_______________________________________________________

_______________________________________________________

_______________________________________________________

_______________________________________________________

_______________________________________________________

_______________________________________________________

# Bonus Weekly Motivation

## Go the Extra Mile

## Your Journey Now Begins

"There are no traffic jams along the extra mile".

-Roger Stauback

## Day Thirty:

Daily Exercise: ______________________________

Calories Burned: ____________________________

Daily Caloric Intake: _________________________

Water Intake: _______________________

Daily Reflections:

________________________________________________________

________________________________________________________

________________________________________________________

________________________________________________________

________________________________________________________

________________________________________________________

________________________________________________________

# Bonus Weekly Motivation

## Go the Extra Mile

## Your Journey Now Begins

"The longest and toughest journeys are normally the most rewarding." -Unknown

## Day Thirty-One:

Daily Exercise: ______________________________

Calories Burned: ____________________________

Daily Caloric Intake: _________________________

Water Intake: ______________________

Daily Reflections:

_______________________________________________________

_______________________________________________________

_______________________________________________________

_______________________________________________________

_______________________________________________________

_______________________________________________________

_______________________________________________________

# About the Author

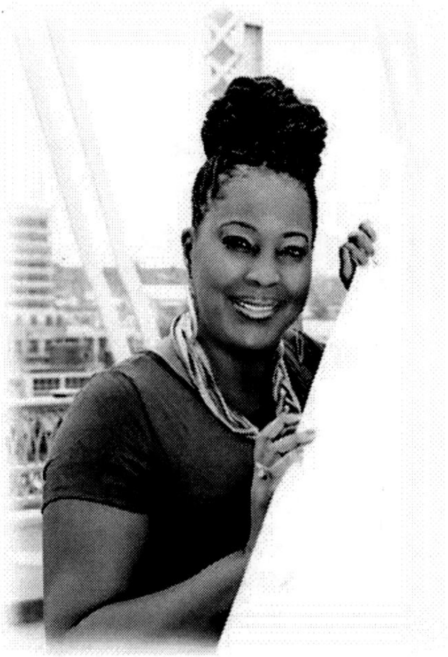

Monica McLaurine has published her first book, in which she shares her inspirational journey to becoming comfortable in her own skin, and living a healthier lifestyle. Her hope is to inspire others to live healthier, and be vigilant in their individual journeys. Most of all, she aspires to ignite others to follow their dreams and position themselves to capture them.

A native of Nashville, Tennessee, Monica has a Bachelor's degree in Criminal Justice, with a concentration with Juvenile Justice from the University of Tennessee at Chattanooga. In her spare time, Monica loves to spend time with family and friends, travel, exercise and shop.